The Complete Calorie Counter

Also in Pan Books

The Complete Carbohydrate Counter
with an introduction by Katie Stewart

compiled by Kyle Cathie
with an introduction by
Eileen Fowler MBE

The complete
calorie counter

Pan Original Pan Books

First published 1976 by Pan Books

This revised edition published 1989 by Pan Books
an imprint of Pan Macmillan Ltd
Pan Macmillan, 20 New Wharf Road, London N1 9RR
Basingstoke and Oxford
Associated companies throughout the world
www.panmacmillan.com

ISBN 0 330 30727 4

29 28 27 26 25 24

A CIP catalogue record for this book is available from
the British Library.

Photoset by Parker Typesetting Service, Leicester
Printed and bound in Great Britain by
Mackays of Chatham PLC, Chatham, Kent

Contents

Introduction
by Eileen Fowler

Sometimes I wonder whether we have the wrong approach to overweight, if we tend to take it for granted that those who suffer from this very contemporary problem are greedy, weak and stupid. I think there are often deep-seated reasons for compulsive eating, that it acts like a drug, and is some form of escapism. But whether the tendencies are inherited or acquired, indulging one's love of food can be extremely dangerous.

This we know, and when excessive weight makes life uncomfortable, we usually do something about it, but it's a great deal easier and safer to control if it's recognized in the early stages. For instance, you hear someone murmur confidentially, 'I'm beginning to get a spare tyre round my waist. It's not what I eat, you know. I cannot understand it: I'm not doing anything different.' But they are – we all are. Times have changed, and as we approach our forties and fifties we tend to take more interest in food and less in exercise.

Take a look around you at your family and friends, and you'll see what I mean. No longer the walk after the evening meal. There's something you want to see on television – anyway there's a car outside if you must go out. Our friends, bless them, ask us to dinner, remembering all our favourite dishes and little weaknesses. Misplaced kindness, but what can you say? Just smile and thank them and slide a little further forward on the bathroom scales.

6

But it isn't good enough, is it? We are jeopardizing our health, our looks and our energy. It's so insidious, this weight gathering: just a few extra calories a month and you are quite a bit heavier by Christmas.

However, our bodies have their own way of paying us back when we over-indulge at the festive season, making sure we know that we've offended. Headaches, indigestion and a bloated feeling leave us in no doubt that a little discretion would have made us feel better and left us a little slimmer. The trouble is the more you eat the more you can eat, and the less you eat the less interested you are in food. All this gets you nowhere. You must eat regularly and according to your needs, but for every good reason under the sun, it should be the right kind of food and the right quantity.

Goodness knows, it isn't always our fault if we have to battle with the bulge. Lots of figure problems are occupational. Think how often we have to stoop, sagging at shoulders and chest: washing-up, ironing, bathing the baby, working at desk or bench. We start with occupational hazards that leave us with slack muscles just asking for a coating of fat. The one-time sportsman, used to much muscular effort, often has time no longer for his regular exercise once he is married: his wife is a good cook – so here we go again.

So why don't we take a good look in that long mirror – all alone, mind, with nobody near enough to say, 'What are you worrying about? I like you that way – you're so cuddly.' Now that's all very well, but do you like yourself that way? It's what matters, because in five years' time you won't be just cuddly, you'll be overweight. Figures don't stay the way you want them to; in most cases they tend to thicken and get set as the years go by and only sensible eating and exercise win the battle against time.

But it's not easy, especially for the men. Giving up smoking, business worries, less time to keep themselves fit make it difficult – just when a young and slim appearance is such an advantage.

What sort of shape is your husband in? You can't force a man to do a bit of good for himself, but you can persuade, drop hints, and quietly nudge him along the right road, and what better example than yourself? The way to a man's heart isn't through his stomach unless it's the right way, especially if he has to face up to business entertainment.

Another fallacy is this 'fat and happy' label. I've seen more than enough hidden tension in the overweight. *Relaxed* and *happy*, *yes* – at least you won't be over-eating or drinking too much to quieten your nerves. If you suffer this way, try walking. Yes, I know you've heard all this before, but have you really tried it? Not a short stroll round the park but walking in the exercise sense. Comfortable shoes, and your arms empty and free to swing make it a pleasure and not a chore.

Don't worry too much about the weather; as it becomes a habit you'll get stronger and better able to face up to a stiff breeze or a summer shower. Avoid north-east winds and a soaking downpour, but be properly equipped, just in case. Even if your surroundings as you walk are not exactly ideal, at least you are making your body work and this is what it needs. You don't age because of what you do in this way, but because of what you don't do. I have this on the highest scientific authority. Walking automatically deepens your breathing, cleanses the bloodstream and make hundreds of muscles move, and the tension gradually lessens. This has been my personal experience and I can thoroughly recommend it.

So what's the answer to it all? I think the answer lies within ourselves. Do we want to keep reasonably slim, healthy and energetic, fit for what we have to do and want to do, or is the price too high to pay? It's as simple as that. You see, I believe that we can achieve anything within reason if we make up our minds that it's all worth while. It's literally a question of mind over matter. Why should we be permanently on the defensive against the gibes of our slimmer acquaintances when we can feel well, happy and confident by counting our calories and seeing that our leisure is active?

Perhaps you are thinking – yes, that's all very well, but how boring. Well, at first, maybe, but not if you've ever experienced or even seen the joy that emanates from those who stop slumping and regain their figure, good posture and one hundred per cent efficiency – to say nothing of the loss of double chins, huge upper arms, and legs and ankles that swell.

Group therapy has many advantages for those who wish to slim, just as attending a Keep Fit class makes the going faster. But not everyone has the time to spare or it may not be convenient. So count your calories at home, at work and play. Let's do it – all of us at the same time – as we read this book.

Best wishes,
Eileen Fowler

The value of calorie counting

Calorie counting is probably the easiest and most popular method of weight control. A calorie is a unit of energy. The body uses up these units of energy, so when you take as many calorific units a day as you use up in energy, your weight should remain constant. However, if your intake is 2,500 and your expenditure is 2,000, you have a calorific excess of 500 units, which, in time, represents something like 50 grammes (2oz) of solid fat. It is very difficult to estimate exactly how much energy we use up during a day. Obviously, someone doing manual labour all day long will use more than a person sitting at an office desk. An average thirty-year-old man needs between 2,500 and 3,500 calorific units a day, whereas a woman will use up only between 1,750 and 2,250. As you grow older, you need fewer calories per day – from about the age of twenty-five.

One of the first things to remember when you go on a diet is that you will lose more weight in the first week than in the subsequent ones, because you should be losing extra liquid from your body as well as breaking down fat. To break down the fat cells in your body (which is how you really lose weight and your shape can change), you need to expend more energy per day than you absorb in calorific units through food. If you eat approximately 250 calories less than you use up, then you should break down 25 grammes (1oz) of solid fat; if the difference is 500 calories, then 50 grammes (2oz) of fat will be used up from your body's store of fat, and so on.

It is unwise to go on a crash diet of bananas and water or grapefruit and boiled eggs or any other diet advocating that you lose 3·5 kilogrammes (8lb) during a week. Not only is it bad for your health generally, so that you become run down (and so more susceptible to minor ailments such as colds and coughs, etc.) but you become very bored with eating the same consistency of food – which means that at the end of the diet, your yearning for a baked potato filled with butter, or half a pound of salted peanuts will be increased. On short diets, too, say for a week or two, most of the weight loss results from dehydration of the body system (losing extra water) so that in fact you have not lost any fat at all. So, when you return to your normal daily diet, absorbing the same amount of fluid, your weight will return to what it was immediately before the diet.

The best way to start reducing your weight is to set a limit on calorific intake for a couple of weeks – if you are a woman, say, 1,500 and if you are a man, say, 2,250. At the end of each week, you should have lost approximately 225 grammes ($\frac{1}{2}$lb). If after two weeks, you find that you have not lost weight, then you obviously use up less energy than the 1,500 or 2,250 calorific units you are taking in – or you are forgetting the odd doughnut you bought by mistake . . . You should try reducing your intake of calories by a further 250 units per day. Or, if you want to lose weight at a faster rate than 225 grammes ($\frac{1}{2}$lb), you could reduce your calorific intake to, say, 1,000 or 1,750, so that you should lose about 675–900 grammes (1$\frac{1}{2}$–2lb) of solid fat per week. A calorific deficit of 1,000 units means that you'll lose 450 grammes (1lb) in four days or about 3·5 kilogrammes (8lb) in a month. You should not enlarge your calorific deficit beyond 1,000 units per day without consulting your doctor.

Each type of food – fat, protein, carbohydrate – converts to solid fat which is stored around the body. Each is essential to a healthy diet. It is unwise, therefore, to cut out all carbohydrates and fats just because they have higher calorie counts, leaving your intake to consist merely of protein such as meat, if you want a well-balanced and healthy diet. Cut down on fatty foods and carbohydrates, but don't exclude them altogether.

There are one or two points worth making about how you spread your calorific intake throughout the day. It is generally thought that one good big meal a day is sufficient, when taken in conjunction with breakfast, tea and a light lunch or dinner, depending on when you have your main meal. Sometimes you may be entertaining friends or going out for a meal and it may be difficult to limit your calorie intake. However, over the week, you can make adjustments so that, say, at weekends you are allowed two or three hundred more calories than on weekdays. But don't have 5,000 calories one day out of a weekly allowance of, say, 7,000 per week and starve yourself for the rest of the period.

Some people tend to want snacks throughout the day – well, it is thought that small meals, taken often, make weight loss easier, and as long as you keep a strict count of all your snacks and make sure they contain the right mixture of carbohydrate, fat and protein, you should be successful.

It is worth bearing in mind that if you have a large meal in the evening, you will be slightly more likely to put on extra pounds than if you have a large meal in the middle of the day; this is because, if you go to bed soon after a big meal,

12

you will have less chance of using up the calories than if you have an afternoon and evening of activity to use up the energy. Even if you stay in bed all day, you still require about 1,000 calorific units.

You will not find it encouraging to rush into the bathroom each morning to find out how much weight you've lost the previous day. It is best to weigh yourself once a week – and if you do it in the morning after you have been to the lavatory, you will be at your lightest. Keep a weekly chart of your progress – this is one of the best encouragements to keep you from breaking the diet. Chart your present weight and the weight you want to reach and fill it in once a week.

This all boils down to one basic factor – *if you want to lose weight you must eat less*, which is the same as saying you must reduce your intake of calories. Keep counting calories, be sensible about it and you should be able to keep to your right weight.

What you should weigh

Obviously this is only an approximate guide and is simply to give you some sort of target to work to. If you weigh yourself without clothes, then deduct about 1 kilogramme (2 lb) from your weight as shown on the chart which follows. These weights are given for men and women over 25; deduct 0·5 kilogramme (1 lb) for each year under 25 if you are between 18 and 24.

Women

Height		Small frame			Medium frame			Large frame		
ft in	cm	st	lb	kg	st	lb	kg	st	lb	kg
4 10	147·5	6	11	43	7	3	46	7	3	50·5
4 11	150	6	13	44	7	6	47	8	2	52
5 0	152·5	7	2	45·5	7	9	48·5	8	5	53
5 1	155	7	5	47	7	12	50	8	8	54·5
5 2	157·5	7	8	48	8	1	51	8	11	56
5 3	160	7	11	49·5	8	4	52·5	9	0	57
5 4	162·5	8	0	51	8	7	54	9	3	58·5
5 5	165	8	4	52·5	8	11	56	9	7	60
5 6	167.5	8	6	53·5	9	1	57·5	9	11	62
5 7	170	8	10	55	9	5	59·5	10	1	64
5 8	172·5	9	0	57	9	9	61	10	5	66
5 9	175	9	4	59	9	13	63	10	9	67·5
5 10	177·5	9	9	61	10	3	65	11	0	70
5 11	180	9	13	63	10	7	67	11	4	71·5
6 0	182·5	10	5	66	10	11	68·5	11	9	74

Men

Height		Small frame			Medium frame			Large frame		
ft in	cm	st	lb	kg	st	lb	kg	st	lb	kg
5 2	157·5	8	4	52·5	8	11	56	9	7	60
5 3	160	8	7	54	9	1	57·5	9	10	61·5
5 4	162·5	8	10	55	9	4	59	10	0	63·5
5 5	165	8	13	57	9	7	60	10	3	65
5 6	167·5	9	2	58	9	10	61·5	10	7	67
5 7	170	9	6	59·5	10	0	63·5	10	11	68·5
5 8	172·5	9	10	61·5	10	5	66	11	2	70·5
5 9	175	10	0	63·5	10	9	67·5	11	6	72·5
5 10	177·5	10	5	66	10	13	69	11	10	74
5 11	180	10	9	67·5	11	3	71	12	1	76·5
6 0	182·5	10	13	69	11	8	73	12	6	79
6 1	185	11	3	71	11	12	75	12	10	80·5
6 2	187·5	11	7	73	12	3	77·5	13	1	83
6 3	190	11	11	75	12	8	80	13	6	85
6 4	192·5	12	1	76·5	12	13	82	13	11	88

Calorie counter

This chart gives the approximate calorific values for 100 grammes and 1 ounce of the particular food. (Both figures have been given to the nearest whole number.)

Note The calorific values calculated for this book are taken from McCance and Widdowson's *The Composition of Foods*, fourth revised and extended edition of MRC Special Report No 297, by A. A. Paul and D. A. T. Southgate, issued by Her Majesty's Stationery Office.

	per 100 g	per oz
Aero	521	147
All–Bran	273	78
Almonds, fresh, shelled	565	161
Alpen	366	104
Angel Delight, chocolate (per sachet made up)	125	36
Angel Delight, raspberry (per sachet made up)	123	35
Apple, baked	31	8
Apple, cooking	37	10
Apple crumble	208	59
Apple, eating	35	10
Apple dumpling	202	57
Apple juice	45	13
Apple pie	369	105
Apple pudding	239	68
Apple, stewed, sweetened	66	19
Apple, stewed, unsweetened	32	9
Apricots, dried	182	52
Apricots, dried, stewed, unsweetened	66	19
Apricots, fresh	28	8
Apricots, stewed, sweetened	60	17
Apricots, stewed, unsweetened	23	6
Apricots, tinned in syrup	106	30
Apricots, tinned in fruit juice	30	9
Arrowroot, powder	355	101
Artichoke, globe, boiled	15	4
Artichoke, Jerusalem, boiled	18	5
Asparagus, boiled	18	5
Aubergine	14	4
Avocado pear, without dressing	223	63

	per 100 g/per oz	
Bacon, back, fried	465	132
Bacon, back, grilled	405	115
Bacon, streaky, fried	496	141
Bacon, streaky, grilled	422	120
Baking powder	163	46
Banana, peeled	79	23
Banana custard	103	29
Barcelona nuts, shelled	639	179
Barley, pearl, raw	360	102
Barley, pearl, boiled	120	29
Barley water, lemon	108	31
Bass, steamed	67	19
Beans, baked, tinned	64	18
Beans, broad, fresh, boiled	48	13
Beans, broad, tinned	55	16
Beans, butter, raw	273	78
Beans, butter, fresh, boiled	95	27
Beans, butter, tinned	90	25
Beans, French, boiled	7	2
Beans, green, runner, boiled	19	5
Beans, green, runner, tinned	10	3
Beans, haricot, boiled	89	25
Beans, red, kidney	272	77
Beans and burgers, tinned	95	27
Beans and sausages, tinned	123	35
Beansprouts	9	3
Beef, mince, stewed	229	65
Beef, rump steak, grilled	218	62
Beef, sirloin, roast	284	81
Beef, stewing steak, stewed	223	63
Beef, topside, roast	214	61

	per 100 g/per oz	
Beef, corned, without sugar	217	62
Beef sausages, fried	269	76
Beef stew	119	34
Beefburgers, fried	264	75
Beefsteak pudding	223	63
Beetroot, boiled	44	13
Bemax	347	99
Bilberries, raw	56	16
Biscuits, Cheddars	554	158
Biscuits, cream crackers	440	125
Biscuits, digest. ⁄e	471	133
Biscuits, digestive, chocolate	493	140
Biscuits, fig roll	350	99
Biscuits, Garibaldi	360	102
Biscuits, ginger snaps	456	130
Biscuits, Hobnobs	493	140
Biscuits, plain	435	123
Biscuits, sponge fingers	400	114
Biscuits, sweet	469	138
Biscuits, Tuc Sandwich	569	162
Biscuits, vanilla wafers	535	151
Biscuits, water	440	125
Blackberries, fresh, unsweetened	29	8
Blackberries, stewed, sweetened	60	17
Blackberries, stewed, unsweetened	25	7
Blackberries, tinned in fruit juice	40	11
Blackberry pie	369	105
Blackcurrants, raw, unsweetened	28	8
Blackcurrants, stewed, sweetened	59	17
Blackcurrants, stewed, unsweetened	24	7
Blackcurrant pie	369	105

	per 100 g/per oz	
Black pudding, fried	305	87
Bloater, grilled	186	53
Boiled sweets	327	93
Bolognese sauce	139	40
Bounty bar	473	134
Bournvita	377	107
Bovril meat extract	174	50
Brains, calves', boiled	152	43
Brains, lambs', boiled	126	36
Bran, wheat	206	58
Brawn	153	43
Brazil nuts, shelled	619	176
Bread, brown	223	63
Bread, currant	250	71
Bread, fried, white	558	158
Bread, Hovis	228	65
Bread, malt	248	70
Bread sauce	110	31
Bread, soda	264	75
Bread, starch-reduced rolls	384	109
Bread, toasted, white	297	84
Bread, white	233	66
Bread, wholemeal	216	61
Bread and butter pudding	159	45
Breadcrumbs, dried	354	100
Bream	66	19
Brill, steamed	78	22
Broccoli, fresh, boiled	18	5
Brown sauce, bottled	99	28
Brussels sprouts, fresh, boiled	26	7
Buck rarebit	287	81

	per 100 g/per oz	
Buns, currant	302	86
Butter	740	213
Butter, peanut, crunchy	613	174
Cabbage, red, raw	20	6
Cabbage, Savoy, boiled	9	3
Cabbage, Savoy, raw	26	7
Canary pudding	461	131
Carrots, new, tinned	19	5
Carrots, old, boiled	19	5
Carrots, old, raw	23	6
Cashew nuts, salted	626	178
Castle pudding	394	112
Catfish, fried in batter	188	53
Cauliflower, fresh, boiled	9	3
Cauliflower, fresh, raw	13	4
Cauliflower cheese	113	32
Celeriac, boiled	14	4
Celery, boiled or braised	5	1
Celery, raw	8	2
Chapatis, made with fat	336	95
Chapatis, made without fat	202	57
Cheese, Camembert	300	85
Cheese, Cheddar	406	115
Cheese, cottage	96	27
Cheese, cream	439	124
Cheese, Danish Blue	355	101
Cheese, Edam	304	86
Cheese, Parmesan	408	116
Cheese, Stilton	462	131

	per 100 g/	per oz
Cheese omelette	170	48
Cheese pudding	170	48
Cheese sauce	198	56
Cheese spread	283	80
Cheese straws	359	102
Cheesecake	421	119
Cherries, fresh, raw	41	11
Cherries, fresh, stewed, sweetened	67	19
Cherries, fresh, stewed, unsweetened	33	9
Cherries, glacé	212	60
Cherry and coconut cake	440	125
Chestnuts, shelled	170	48
Chicken, boiled	183	52
Chicken, roast	148	42
Chicken, wing	74	21
Chicken, leg	92	26
Chicken curry	160	46
Chicken pie	275	78
Chicken soup, tinned	58	16
Chicken spread	220	63
Chicken supreme, tinned	159	45
Chicken and ham pie	235	67
Chicken and noodle soup mix, made up	20	6
Chicory, raw	9	3
Chocolate biscuits	524	148
Chocolate cup cakes	335	95
Chocolate, drinking, powder	366	104
Chococlate, fancy	460	131
Chocolate, fruit and nut	495	141
Chocolate, milk	529	150
Chocolate mousse (Chambourcy)	197	56

	per 100 g/per oz	
Chocolate, plain	525	149
Chocolate pudding	296	84
Chocolate, whole nut	560	159
Christmas pudding	304	86
Chutney, apple	193	55
Chutney, tomato	154	44
Cob nuts, shelled	380	108
Coca-cola	39	11
Cockles	48	13
Cocoa, powder	312	89
Coconut, desiccated	604	171
Coconut, fresh	351	100
Coconut milk	21	6
Cod, baked	82	23
Cod, fillets, frozen	68	19
Cod, fried in batter	199	57
Cod, grilled	95	27
Cod, roe, baked in vinegar	128	37
Cod, roe, fried	202	57
Cod liver oil	899	260
Coffee, black, made up	2	1
Coffee and chicory essence	218	62
Coleslaw	110	31
Conger eel, stewed	201	57
Cooking fat	894	259
Corn oil	899	260
Corn on the cob	123	35
Corned beef	217	62
Cornflakes	368	104
Cornflour	354	100
Cornish pasties	332	95

	per 100 g/per oz	
Cottage pie	119	34
Crab, boiled	127	36
Cranberries, fresh	15	4
Cream, fresh, double	447	127
Cream, fresh, single	212	60
Cream, fresh, whipping	332	95
Cream, whipping, longlife	330	94
Cream, soured	180	51
Cream, tinned, single	230	65
Cream, top of the milk	212	60
Cream, imitation	110	31
Crispbread, wheat, starch-reduced	388	110
Crispbread, rye	321	91
Crisps, potato	533	151
Crumpets	175	50
Crunchie bar (per bar)	195	55
Cucumber, raw	10	3
Currant buns	302	86
Currant cake	418	119
Curried meat	160	46
Curry powder	233	66
Custard, baked egg	118	34
Custard powder, made up	118	34
Custard powder, raw	354	100
Custard tart	287	82
Dabs, fried	199	56
Damsons, fresh, raw	34	9
Damsons, fresh, stewed, sweetened	63	18
Damsons, fresh, stewed, unsweetened	29	8
Dates, fresh, weighed with stones	214	61

	per 100 g/per oz	
Dates, dried, stoned	248	70
Dogfish, fried	300	85
Doughnuts	349	99
Dripping, beef	891	258
Duck, roast	339	96
Dumplings	211	60
Dundee cake	389	110
Easter biscuit	473	134
Eccles cakes	518	147
Eclairs	376	107
Eels	201	57
Eggs, boiled	147	42
Eggs, fried	232	66
Eggs, poached	155	44
Eggs, scrambled	246	70
Egg sauce	148	42
Egg, Scotch	279	79
Endive	11	3
Faggots	268	76
Farex	348	97
Figs, dried, raw	213	61
Figs, dried, stewed, sweetened	136	39
Figs, dried, stewed, unsweetened	118	34
Figs, fresh	41	12
Fish cakes, fried	188	53
Fish fingers, fried	233	66
Fish paste	169	48
Flake (per bar)	170	48
Flounder, fried	147	42
Flounder, steamed or grilled	53	15

	per 100 g	per oz
Flour, wholemeal (100%)	318	90
Flour, brown (85%)	327	93
Flour, white (72%), breadmaking	337	96
Flour, household, plain	350	101
Flour, self-raising	339	96
Flour, Manitoba, patent (40%)	347	99
Frankfurter	274	78
French dressing	658	186
Fruit cake, rich	332	95
Fruit cake, rich, iced	352	100
Fruit gums	172	49
Fruit pie, individual, pastry	369	105
Fruit salad, tinned in syrup	95	27
Fruit salad, tinned in fruit juice	40	11
Fudge	422	120
Gammon, boiled	269	76
Ginger biscuits	456	130
Ginger, ground	258	74
Gingerbread	373	106
Glucose	318	90
Goose	173	49
Gooseberries, fresh	17	5
Gooseberries, stewed, sweetened	50	14
Gooseberries, stewed, unsweetened	14	4
Gooseberries, tarts	369	105
Gooseberry pie	369	105
Grape juice, red	60	17
Grape juice, white	55	16
Grapefruit, fresh, unsweetened	11	3
Grapefruit juice, tinned, sweetened	38	11

	per 100 g/per oz	
Grapefruit juice, tinned, unsweetened	31	9
Grapefruit squash, concentrated	136	39
Grapefruit, tinned	60	17
Grapenuts	355	101
Grapes, black, fresh	51	14
Grapes, green, fresh	60	17
Greengages, fresh, unstoned	45	13
Greengages, stewed, sweetened	75	21
Greengages, stewed, unsweetened	40	11
Grouse, roast	114	32
Guinea fowl, roast	114	32
Haddock, fried	160	46
Haddock, smoked	66	19
Haddock, steamed	75	21
Haggis	310	88
Hake, fried	193	55
Hake, steamed	86	24
Halibut, steamed	99	28
Ham	120	34
Ham and pork, chopped loaf	270	77
Hare, stewed	192	54
Hazel nuts, shelled	380	108
Heart, ox, stewed	179	51
Heart, sheep, roast	237	67
Herring, fried	206	58
Herring, grilled	135	38
Herring roe, fried	244	69
Honey	288	82
Honeycomb	281	80
Horlicks powder	396	113

	per 100 g/per oz	
Horseradish, raw	59	17
Hot-pot, Lancashire	114	32
Ice-cream, dairy	167	48
Ice-cream, non-dairy	165	47
Instant Whip, fruit, made up	358	102
Irish stew	124	35
Jaffa juice, orange squash, tinned	33	9
Jam, generally	261	74
Jam, reduced sugar	125	36
Jam roll (Swiss)	360	102
Jam tarts	384	109
Jelly, raw, fruit	259	74
Jelly, made up	59	17
Jelly, milk	86	24
John Dory, steamed	59	17
Kedgeree	151	43
Ketchup, tomato	98	28
Kidney, lamb, fried	155	44
Kidney, ox, stewed	172	49
Kidney, pig, stewed	153	43
Kippers	111	31
KitKat (per bar)	245	69
Lamb, chop, grilled	355	101
Lamb, cutlet, grilled	370	105
Lamb, leg, roast	266	75
Lamb, scrag and neck, stewed	292	83
Lamb, shoulder, roast	316	90

	per 100 g/per oz	
Lard	891	252
Laverbread	52	15
Leeks, boiled	24	7
Leeks, raw	31	9
Lemon, fresh	15	4
Lemon barley water, concentrated	108	31
Lemon curd, homemade	290	82
Lemon curd, starch based	283	80
Lemon curd tarts	442	125
Lemon juice, fresh	7	2
Lemon meringue pie	323	92
Lemon sole, steamed	64	18
Lemon sole, fried	171	49
Lemonade	21	6
Lentils, boiled	99	28
Lentils, dried, uncooked	304	86
Lentil soup	99	28
Lettuce	12	4
Lime juice cordial, undiluted	112	32
Ling, fried	185	52
Lion Bar (per bar)	240	68
Liquorice all-sorts	313	89
Liver, calf, fried	254	72
Liver, chicken, fried	194	55
Liver, lamb, fried	232	66
Liver, ox, stewed	198	56
Liver, pig's, stewed	189	54
Liver sausage	310	88
Lobster, boiled	119	34
Loganberries, raw	17	5
Loganberries, stewed, sweetened	54	15

	per 100 g/per oz	
Loganberries, stewed, unsweetened	16	5
Loganberries, tinned in syrup	101	29
Low fat spread	366	104
Lucozade	68	19
Luncheon meat	313	89
Lychees, fresh	64	18
Lychees, tinned	68	19
Macaroni, boiled	117	33
Macaroni cheese	174	50
Macaroni cheese, tinned	106	30
Macaroni, raw	370	105
Mackerel, fried	138	39
Madeira cake	393	111
Maltesers	478	135
Mandarins, tinned	56	16
Mango, fresh	59	17
Mango, tinned	77	22
Margarine (all kinds)	730	210
Marmalade	261	74
Marmalade, reduced sugar	125	36
Marmite	179	51
Marrow, boiled	7	2
Mars bar	441	125
Marvel, milk powder	355	101
Marzipan	443	126
Mayonnaise	718	208
Meat balls, in gravy	81	23
Meat paste	173	49
Medlars	42	12
Melon, cantaloup	15	4

	per 100 g/per oz	
Melon, honeydew	13	4
Melon, watermelon	11	3
Meringues	380	108
Milk, fresh, dairy	65	18
Milk, condensed, full cream, sweetened	322	92
Milk, condensed, skimmed, sweetened	267	76
Milk, evaporated, unsweetened	158	45
Milk powder, full cream	490	139
Milk powder, low fat	355	101
Milk, skimmed	33	9
Mincemeat	235	67
Mince pies	435	123
Minestrone, dried mix, made up	23	7
Minstrels	500	142
Mints, After Eight Thin	409	116
Mints, glacier (Fox's)	371	106
Mixed fruit pudding	325	92
Mixed peel, candied	255	72
Molasses	257	73
Monkfish, fried	145	41
Monkfish, steamed or grilled	79	23
Moussaka	195	55
Muesli	368	105
Mulberries	36	10
Mullet, red or grey, steamed	85	24
Mushrooms, fried	210	60
Mushrooms, raw	13	4
Mushroom soup, tinned	53	15
Mussels, boiled	87	25
Mustard and cress, raw	10	3
Mustard powder	452	128

	per 100 g/per oz	
Nectarines	46	13
Nescafé, black, made up	0	0
Nescafé, powder	100	28
Oatcakes	441	125
Oatmeal porridge, boiled	44	13
Oil, cooking, olive and vegetable	899	260
Okra	17	5
Olives, black and green	82	23
Omelette, plain	190	54
Onion, boiled	13	4
Onion, fried	345	98
Onion, raw	23	6
Onion sauce	99	28
Onion, spring	35	10
Orange, fresh, whole	26	7
Orange cake, plain	465	132
Orange juice, fresh	38	11
Orange juice, tinned, unsweetened	33	9
Orange squash, concentrated	107	30
Outline low-calorie fat spread	370	105
Ovaltine, powder	376	107
Oxo cubes	229	65
Oxtail, stewed	92	26
Oxtail soup, tinned	44	13
Ox tongue, pickled	293	83
Oysters, raw	51	14
Pancakes	307	87
Parsley, fresh	21	6
Parsnip, boiled	56	16

	per 100 g/per oz	
Parsnip, raw	49	14
Partridge, roast	127	36
Passion fruit	14	4
Pasta, lasagne, uncooked	325	92
Pasta, quill, cooked	140	40
Pasta, quill, uncooked	340	96
Pasta, rigatoni, uncooked	325	92
Pasta, shells, cooked	155	44
Pasta, shells, uncooked	340	96
Pasta, spaghetti, cooked	110	31
Pasta, wholewheat instant spirals, uncooked	340	96
Pastilles	253	72
Pastry, choux, baked	330	94
Pastry, flaky, baked	565	161
Pastry, shortcrust, baked	527	149
Pâté	465	132
Pawpaw, tinned	65	18
Peach, fresh	32	9
Peach, dried	212	60
Peach, dried, stewed, unsweetened	79	23
Peach, stewed, sweetened	93	26
Peach, tinned in syrup	87	24
Peach, tinned in fruit juice	35	10
Peanut butter, smooth	623	177
Peanuts, shelled, salted	570	162
Pear, fresh	29	8
Pear, stewed, sweetened	65	18
Pear, stewed, unsweetened	30	8
Pear, tinned in syrup	77	22
Pear, tinned in fruit juice	35	10

	per 100 g/	per oz
Peas, dried, boiled	103	29
Peas, fresh, boiled	52	15
Peas, fresh, raw	67	19
Peas, frozen, boiled	41	12
Peas, split, boiled	118	34
Peas, tinned, garden	47	13
Peas, tinned, processed	80	23
Pease pudding	85	24
Pepper, black or white	308	87
Peppers, red or green	15	4
Peppermints	392	111
Pheasant, roast	134	38
Pickle, mustard (Heinz)	114	32
Pickle, piccalilli	33	9
Pickle, ploughman's (Heinz)	120	34
Pickle, sweet	134	38
Pickle, tomato (Heinz)	95	27
Pigeon, roast	101	29
Pilchard, tinned in tomato sauce	126	36
Pineapple, fresh, weighed with skin	46	13
Pineapple juice, tinned	53	15
Pineapple, tinned in syrup	77	22
Pineapple, tinned in juice	61	17
Pizza	234	66
Plaice, steamed	50	14
Plaice, fried in batter	279	79
Plaice, fried and breadcrumbed	228	65
Plantain, boiled	122	35
Plantain, fried	267	76
Plums, fresh, dessert, unstoned	36	10
Plums, cooking, stewed, sweetened	55	16

	per 100 g/per oz	
Plums, cooking, stewed, unsweetened	20	6
Plums, pie	369	105
Plums, tinned	70	20
Pollack, steamed or grilled	58	16
Pollack, fried in batter	145	41
Polony	281	80
Pork, belly, grilled	398	113
Pork, chop, grilled	332	95
Pork, leg, roast	286	81
Pork pie	376	107
Porridge, made up	44	13
Porridge instant oats	401	114
Potato, baked	85	24
Potato, boiled, new	76	22
Potato, boiled, old	80	23
Potato, chipped, frozen	291	83
Potato, chipped, old	253	72
Potato crisps	533	151
Potato, instant, made up	70	20
Potato, mashed	119	34
Potato, roast, old	157	45
Potato soup	92	26
Potato, tinned, new	53	15
Prawns	107	30
Prunes, dried, unstoned	134	38
Prunes, dried, stewed, unsweetened	74	21
Prunes, tinned in syrup	95	27
Puffed Wheat	325	92
Pumpkin	15	4

	per 100g/per oz	
Quaker Oats, raw	401	114
Queen cakes	455	129
Queen of Puddings	216	61
Quiche Lorraine	391	111
Quince, fresh	25	7
Rabbit, stewed	91	26
Radish, raw	15	4
Raisins, dried	246	70
Raisins, dried, seedless	247	70
Raspberries, fresh	25	7
Raspberries, stewed, sweetened	68	19
Raspberries, stewed, unsweetened	26	7
Raspberries, tinned in syrup	87	24
Ravioli, tinned	75	21
Ready Brek	390	111
Red currants	21	6
Rhubarb, fresh, stewed, sweetened	45	13
Rhubarb, fresh, stewed, unsweetened	6	2
Rhubarb pie	369	105
Rhubarb, tinned in syrup	30	8
Ribena, concentrated	229	65
Ribena, diluted	188	53
Rice, boiled	123	35
Rice, creamed	90	25
Rice pudding, tinned	91	26
Rice, raw	361	74
Rice Krispies	372	77
Rock cakes	394	112
Roe, cod's, fried	202	57
Rosehip syrup, concentrated	232	66

	per 100 g/per oz	
Rye flour (100%)	335	95
Ryvita	317	90
Sago, raw	355	101
Sago, creamed, tinned	91	26
Sago pudding	131	37
Saithe, steamed	84	24
Salad cream	311	88
Salad dressing	658	186
Salami	491	139
Salmon, smoked	142	40
Salmon, steamed	160	46
Salmon, tinned	155	44
Salsify, boiled	18	5
Salt	0	0
Sardines, tinned in oil	217	62
Sausages, pork, fried	317	90
Sausages, beef, fried	269	76
Sausages, black	305	87
Sausage, liver	310	88
Sausages, luncheon meat	313	89
Sausages, rolls	479	136
Saveloy	262	74
Scallops	105	30
Scampi, boiled	117	33
Scampi, fried	316	90
Scones	371	106
Scotch broth, tinned	55	16
Scotch egg	279	79
Scotch pancakes	283	80
Seakale, boiled	8	2

	per 100 g/	per oz
Semolina, raw	350	99
Semolina, creamed	109	31
Semolina pudding	131	37
Shepherd's pie	119	34
Shortbread	504	144
Shredded Wheat	324	92
Shreddies	330	94
Shrimps, boiled	117	33
Skate, fried in batter	163	46
Smarties	173	49
Smelts, fried	346	98
Sole, lemon, fried	171	49
Sole, lemon, steamed	64	18
Soya flour, full fat	447	127
Soya flour, low fat	352	106
Spaghetti, raw	378	108
Spaghetti, cooked, plain	117	33
Spaghetti Bolognese, tinned	346	98
Spaghetti, tinned, with tomato sauce	59	17
Special K	388	111
Spinach, fresh, boiled	30	8
Sponge cake, made with fat	464	132
Sponge cake, made without fat	301	86
Sponge cake, with jam	302	86
Sponge pudding, steamed	344	98
Sprats, fried	388	111
Spring greens, boiled	10	3
St Ivel Gold	390	111
Steak, rump, grilled	218	62
Steak, stewed with gravy	176	50
Steak and kidney pie	286	81

	per 100 g/per oz	
Stock cubes	229	65
Strawberries, fresh	26	7
Strawberries, tinned in syrup	81	23
Stuffing, country	365	104
Sturgeon, steamed	105	30
Suet	895	259
Suet, shredded	826	233
Suet pudding	333	95
Sugar, all kinds	394	112
Sugar Puffs	348	99
Sultanas	250	71
Swedes, boiled	18	5
Sweetbreads, fried	230	65
Sweetcorn, on-the-cob, boiled	123	35
Sweetcorn, tinned	76	22
Sweet potatoes, boiled	85	24
Syrup, golden	298	85
Syrup, golden, pudding	288	82
Tangerines, fresh, weighed with skins	23	6
Tapioca, raw	359	102
Tapioca pudding	131	37
Tartare sauce	282	80
Tea, without milk	0	0
Toad-in-the-hole	290	82
Toast, white	297	84
Toffee	430	122
Toffee Crisp (per bar)	243	69
Tomato, fresh, raw	14	4
Tomato, fresh, fried	69	19
Tomato juice, tinned	16	5

	per 100 g	per oz
Tomato ketchup	98	28
Tomato purée	67	19
Tomato sauce	86	24
Tomato soup, tinned	55	16
Tomatoes, tinned	12	4
Tongue, sheep, stewed	289	82
Tongue, ox, pickled	293	83
Topic (per bar)	232	66
Treacle, black	257	73
Treacle pudding	288	82
Treacle tart	371	106
Trifle	160	46
Tripe, stewed	100	28
Trout, steamed	89	25
Tuna, tinned in oil	289	82
Turbot, steamed	66	19
Turkey, roast	171	49
Turkish delight (Fry's), per bar	180	51
Turnips, boiled	14	4
Turnip tops, boiled	11	3
Veal, cutlets, fried	215	61
Veal, fillet, roast	230	65
Vegetable oil	899	260
Vegetable soup, tinned	37	11
Venison, roast	197	56
Victoria sandwich	302	86
Vinegar	4	1
Virol	349	99
Vita-Weat	423	120

	per 100 g/per oz	
Walnuts, shelled	525	149
Watercress, fresh	14	4
Weetabix	340	96
Welsh cheesecakes	489	139
Welsh rarebit	365	104
Whelks	91	26
Whitebait, fried	525	149
Whiting, fried	173	49
Whiting, steamed or boiled	63	18
White sauce, savoury	151	43
White sauce, sweet	172	49
Winkles	74	21
Wispa (per bar)	195	55
Witch, fried	196	56
Witch, steamed or boiled	53	15
Yams, boiled	119	34
Yeast, baker's	53	15
Yeast, dried	169	48
Yoghurt, natural	52	15
Yoghurt, flavoured	81	23
Yoghurt, fruit	95	27
Yoghurt, hazelnut	106	30
Yorkshire pudding	215	60

Alcoholic drinks

All measurements are either standard can sizes or standard pub measurements.

Beer	approx per pint	per fl oz	per 100 ml
Brown ale, bottled	160	8	28
Canned beer, bitter	180	9	32
Draught ale, bitter	180	9	32
Draught ale, mild	140	7	25
Keg bitter	180	9	31
Lager, bottled	160	8	29
Pale ale, bottled	180	9	32
Stout, bottled	200	10	37
Stout, extra	220	11	39
Strong ale	420	21	72

Cider			
Dry	200	10	36
Sweet	240	12	42
Vintage	560	28	101

Wines	approx per glass		
Port, ruby	129	43	152
Port, tawny	135	45	160
Rosé	100	20	71
Sherry, dry	99	33	115
Sherry, medium	102	34	118
Sherry, sweet	114	38	136
Champagne	106	21	76

	approx per glass	per fl oz	per 100 ml
Graves	105	21	73
Sauternes	130	26	94
Burgundy	100	20	72
Beaujolais	95	19	68
Chianti	90	18	65
Médoc	90	18	63

Spirits

Spirits	per pub measure $\frac{1}{6}$th gill
Scotch whisky	58
Irish whiskey	63
Gin	55
Rum	75
Vodka	63

Soft drinks

Soft drinks	12 oz tin	per fl oz	per 100 ml
Coca-cola		11	39
Tab	·75	—	—
Lucozade		19	68
Bitter lemon		9	32
Dry ginger ale		4	14
Ginger beer		11	39
American ginger ale		11	39
Soda-water		—	—
Tonic water		6	21

Liqueurs

Liqueurs	approx per glass
Benedictine	75
Brandy	75
Chartreuse	75
Cherry brandy	90
Crème de menthe	90
Curaçao	70
Drambuie	65
Kümmel	70

Low-calorie recipes

Starters

Soups can be divided into two groups: thin soups made with home-made stock and which contain no thickening ingredients such as cornflour or potato; and those which contain cream, egg yolks, flour or potatoes. Soups in the second category usually contain a large number of calories per portion and should be avoided by the calorie conscious; I will give some recipes for the first group.

Tomato soup

serves 4   calories per portion: 40

450 g (1 lb) tomatoes	1 tablespoon olive oil
1 large onion, finely sliced	600 ml (1 pint) chicken stock
1 clove garlic, crushed	salt and pepper to taste

Heat the oil in a large saucepan. Add the onion and garlic and fry until softened. Put the tomatoes in boiling water for thirty seconds, then remove the skins. Chop roughly and add to saucepan. Cook for 5 minutes over a low heat and then add the stock. Simmer for 15–20 minutes until the tomatoes are soft, then blend in an electric blender or put through a Mouli. Season with salt and pepper and serve piping hot, garnished with parsley or thin slices of lemon. This soup can also be served cold, in which case it should be chilled in the refrigerator for several hours.

Watercress soup

serves 4   calories per portion: 39

1 onion, finely sliced
2 bunches watercress
600 ml (1 pint) stock
300 ml (½ pint) milk made with 25 g (1 oz) dried low-fat
   milk and 300 ml (½ pint) water
salt and pepper to taste
pinch nutmeg

Wash watercress and remove any tough stalks. Chop
roughly and reserve about half a bunch for decoration at
the end. Put watercress, onion and stock into a large
saucepan and bring to the boil. Simmer gently for 15–20
minutes, until the vegetables are tender. Stir in the milk,
and put through a Mouli or blend in an electric blender.
Adjust seasoning, add nutmeg and serve garnished with
remaining watercress. Serve hot or put in the refrigerator
to chill for several hours.

Consommé with yoghurt and lumpfish roe

serves 3   calories per portion: 55

1 tin Cross & Blackwell's Consommé
1 small carton natural yoghurt
1 small pot Danish lumpfish roe
salt and pepper to taste

In a saucepan, gently heat the consommé until melted.
Season with salt and pepper and pour into individual
bowls. Put in refrigerator to set – this should take one to
two hours. Cover each portion with the yoghurt and then
sprinkle about 1 teaspoon of lumpish roe evenly over the
yoghurt.

Melon balls with orange

serves 4   calories per portion: 65

1 ripe honeydew melon
juice and grated rind of 1 orange
juice of ½ lemon

Cut the melon in half and remove the seeds. Using a round vegetable scoop, cut the melon into round balls. Put them into a large bowl, and mix in the fruit juices and grated orange rind. Allow to chill for several hours and serve in individual bowls.

Moules marinière

serves 4   calories per portion: 60

Mussels are very cheap when in season (roughly from September until April), and although they take a considerable time to clean they do have a reasonably low calorific value.

1 gallon mussels
1 tablespoon olive oil
1 onion, finely sliced
1 clove garlic, crushed
600 ml (1 pint) stock

Clean the mussels and remove the beards. Discard any which are open or which feel very heavy – they may contain mud. Rinse them two or three times in cold water. In a large saucepan, heat the oil and add the onion and garlic. Fry gently until softened and pour in the stock. Bring to the boil and add the mussels. Shake the pan and leave to boil vigorously for 2–3 minutes, by which time the mussels should have opened. Serve in soup bowls with the liquid. Any mussels which have not opened during the cooking stage should be discarded.

Salads and main courses

Salade niçoise

serves 4   calories per portion: 85

2 hard-boiled eggs
2 ripe tomatoes
8 good lettuce leaves
8–10 anchovy fillets

8–10 black olives, stoned
50g (2oz) tuna fish
4 tablespoons vinegar
or lemon juice

Shell the eggs and cut them into quarters. Put the tomatoes in boiling water for 30 seconds and remove the skins. Slice thinly. Arrange the lettuce leaves on four plates, then the eggs and tomatoes. Flake the well-drained tuna fish, arrange on the salads, decorate with the anchovy fillets and olives and pour over the vinegar or lemon juice.

Cottage cheese and cucumber salad

serves 4   calories per portion: 75

225g (8oz) cottage cheese
1 cucumber, finely diced
8–10 black olives, stoned
8 good lettuce leaves
4 tablespoons vinegar or lemon juice
salt and pepper to taste
2 tablespoons chives

In a bowl, mix the cottage cheese with the cucumber and chives. Season with salt and pepper. Arrange the lettuce leaves on four plates, and put a quarter of the mixture on each plate. Decorate with the olives and pour over the dressing of vinegar or lemon juice.

Broad bean and anchovy salad

serves 4   calories per portion: 101

225 g (8 oz) young broad beans
8–10 anchovy fillets
3 hard–boiled eggs
2 tablespoons chives, finely chopped
150 ml (¼ pint) tomato juice
1 tablespoon lemon juice
salt and pepper to taste
8 good lettuce leaves

Cook the broad beans in boiling salted water until tender.
Drain and leave to cool. Shell the eggs and cut into
quarters. Arrange lettuce leaves, broad beans and eggs on
four separate plates. Mix the tomato juice, lemon juice and
salt and pepper well and pour over the salads. Sprinkle
with chives.

Eggs with spinach

serves 4   calories per portion: 115

450 g (1 lb) spinach
4 eggs
salt and pepper to taste

Wash the spinach and discard any tough leaves. Boil it in a
large saucepan with 150 ml (¼ pint) water for 15 minutes or
until tender, and drain well. Put the spinach into a large
ovenproof dish, shape four holes in it and break an egg into
each hole. Put it into a pre-heated oven (175°C, 350°F, Gas
4) for about 10 minutes or until the eggs are just set. Season
with salt and pepper and serve.

Savoury tomatoes

serves 4   calories per portion: 110

4 large tomatoes
50 g (2 oz) cold meat (ham or chicken)
1 small onion, finely sliced
50 g (2 oz) grated Cheddar cheese
salt and pepper to taste

Cut the tops off the tomatoes, scoop out the insides and mix them in a bowl with the finely chopped cold meat and the onion. Add the cheese and season. Spoon the mixture back into the tomatoes, replace the tops and bake in a moderate oven (175°C, 350°F, Gas 4) for 30 minutes.

Kedgeree

serves 3   calories per portion: 287

225 g (8 oz) smoked haddock, steamed
50 g (2 oz) rice
25 g (1 oz) margarine
1 hard-boiled egg
1 egg
salt and pepper to taste

Boil the rice in 1½ cupfuls of salted water for 15 minutes or until cooked. Drain and add to another saucepan in which you have melted the margarine. Add the flaked fish, the egg, beaten, and season with salt and pepper. Mix well and add the chopped hard-boiled egg. Turn the mixture into a well-greased pie dish and bake in a moderate oven (175°C, 350°F, Gas 4) for 20 minutes.

Grilled steak with lemon

serves 2   calories per portion: 328

2 steaks, approximately 170g (6oz) each
25g (1oz) margarine
freshly ground black pepper
½ lemon

Trim any excess fat off the steaks and season them with pepper. Heat the grill until really hot. Lay the steaks on the grill rack, dot with margarine and grill for 3–8 minutes on each side depending on how rare you like them. Serve with quarters of lemon.

Grilled trout with lemon

serves 2   calories per portion: 154

2 trout, approximately 340g (12oz) each
salt and freshly ground black pepper
1 tablespoon parsley, finely chopped
½ lemon

Clean the fish, slit open and remove the innards. Whether you leave the head on or not is up to you; some people are put off by it and others think it makes the fish look better. Cut two or three gashes in the sides of the fish to allow the heat to get through to the bone. Season both the inside and outside of the fish and put under a hot grill for about 6–7 minutes on each side. Decorate the wounds of the fish with parsley and serve piping hot with quarters of lemon.

Beef casserole

serves 4   calories per portion: 424

25 g (1 oz) butter
1 onion, finely sliced
1 clove garlic, crushed
450 g (1 lb) stewing steak
600 ml (1 pint) good stock
50 g (2 oz) mushrooms
450 g (1 lb) carrots
salt and pepper

Melt half the butter in a large pan, add the onion and garlic and cook until soft. Add the meat, cut up into small cubes and continue to cook until the meat is browned on all sides. Peel the carrots, slice lengthwise and add to the pan, together with the stock. Cook in a moderate oven (160°C, 325°F, Gas 3) for about 1½ hours. Remove pan and add sliced mushrooms that have previously been cooked into the remaining butter. Return pan to oven and continue to cook for half an hour or until the meat is fork-tender. Adjust seasoning and serve.

Vegetable pie

serves 3   calories per portion: 204

100 g (4 oz) mushrooms
2 large onions, finely sliced
white of 1 leek, finely shredded
2 large aubergines, cut into slices
225 g (8 oz) tomatoes
salt and pepper to taste
25 g (1 oz) butter
2 tablespoons water

Sprinkle the aubergine slices with salt and allow to sweat for half an hour. Drain well on kitchen paper. Stand the tomatoes in boiling water for thirty seconds, then remove the skins. Slice them and the mushrooms. Lightly grease a casserole, line it with aubergine slices, followed by layers of mushroom, tomato, leek and onion. Repeat until all the ingredients are used up, finishing with a layer of aubergine. Sprinkle with the cheese, dot with butter and add the water. Bake in a moderate oven (175°C, 350°F, Gas 4) for 1–1½ hours.

Chicken casserole

serves 4   calories per portion: 365

50 g (2 oz) butter
1 large onion, finely sliced
1 clove garlic, crushed
1 chicken, approximately 1 kg (2¼ lb)
1 tablespoonful chopped tarragon
100 g (4 oz) mushrooms
600 ml (1 pint) chicken stock
1 small glass white wine
salt and pepper to taste

Melt half the butter in a frying pan, add the onions and garlic and fry until softened but not brown. Transfer to casserole dish. Add remaining butter to frying pan and add chicken, cut up into joints. Brown on all sides, and put into casserole dish. Pour over stock, white wine, tarragon and season with salt and pepper. Put into a moderate oven (175°C, 350°F, Gas 4) for 1 hour. Remove and add mushrooms. Continue to cook for a further 30 minutes or until the meat is fork-tender.

Cabbage leaves stuffed with minced meat

serves 4   calories per portion: 209

450 g (1 lb) minced meat
1 large onion, finely chopped
1 clove garlic, crushed
1 tablespoon chopped parsley
8 large or 12 small cabbage leaves
300 ml ($\frac{1}{2}$ pint) chicken stock
salt and pepper to taste

Wash the cabbage leaves and boil them in lightly salted water for about five minutes. While you are doing this, mix the meat, onion, garlic and parsley in a large bowl and season well. Drain the cabbage leaves and fill them with the meat mixture. Roll them up and secure each with a cocktail stick. Place in a lightly greased baking dish and pour over the stock. Bake in a moderate oven (175°C, 350°F, Gas 4) for forty-five minutes.

Puddings

Raspberry mousse

serves 4   calories per portion: 110

450 g (1 lb) raspberries
liquid sweetener to taste
2 tablespoons water
4 egg whites

In a large saucepan, boil the raspberries with the sweetener
and water until pulpy – about five minutes. Put them
through a Mouli or blend in an electric blender, to make a
purée. Whisk the egg whites stiff and fold them into the
fruit. Reserve a few raspberries to decorate. Chill for
several hours.

Spiced oranges

serves 4   calories per portion: 50

4 large oranges
450 ml (¾ pint) water
½ teaspoon ground cinnamon
¼ teaspoon freshly ground nutmeg
liquid sweetener

Peel the oranges and remove all the white pith. Cut them
into slices. In a saucepan, heat the water and spices until
boiling point and add the orange slices. Simmer very
gently for three to four minutes. Add liquid sweetener if
desired. Leave to cool, then chill in the refrigerator for
several hours.

Pears in red wine

serves 4   calories per portion: 90

4 large ripe pears
½ teaspoon ground cinnamon
½ teaspoon freshly ground nutmeg
liquid sweetener
450 ml (¾ pint) red cooking wine

Peel the pears, leaving the stalks on and the pears whole. In a large saucepan, heat the spices, 3–4 drops of liquid sweetener and the red wine to boiling point. Add the pears and leave to simmer very gently for 30–45 minutes until the pears are tender. Either serve hot or allow to cool and chill in the refrigerator for several hours.

Rhubarb crumble

serves 4   calories per portion: 190

675 g (1½ lb) rhubarb	25 g (1 oz) butter
3–4 tablespoons water	50 g (2 oz) sugar
liquid sweetener	75 g (3 oz) flour

Cut the rhubarb into 2·5 cm (1 in) slices and put into a saucepan with the water and 3–4 drops of sweetener. You may need more depending on how sweet you like your rhubarb. Bring to the boil and then heat as low as possible, or cook in the oven (140°C, 275°F, Gas 1), covered with a lid, for about fifteen minutes. Pour into a lightly greased ovenproof dish. Make the crumble by mixing the butter, sugar and flour until the butter is all broken down. Put the mixture on top of the rhubarb (if the rhubarb seems very liquid, remove some of the juice). Bake in a moderate oven (175°C, 350°F, Gas 4) for 15–20 minutes by which time the top should be lightly browned. There should be just enough crumble for everyone to have a taste.

Apple meringue

serves 4   calories per portion: 107

675 g (1½ lb) cooking apples
3–4 tablespoons water
liquid sweetener
4 egg whites

Peel and core the apples. Cut them into slices and place in a saucepan with the water and liquid sweetener. Bring to the boil and simmer very gently for 20–30 minutes, then pour into a lightly greased ovenproof dish. Add a few drops of sweetener to the egg whites and beat them until stiff. Cover the apple with the beaten egg whites and bake in a cool oven (150°C, 300°F, Gas 2) for about twenty minutes.

Blackberry fool

serves 4   calories per portion: 70

450 g (1 lb) ripe blackberries
3–4 tablespoons water
liquid sweetener
2 small cartons natural yoghurt

Wash the blackberries well and cook in a large saucepan with the water and a few drops of liquid sweetener for about 8–10 minutes or until tender. Put through an electric blender or Mouli to form a pulp. Test for sweetness and add more sweetener if necessary. Allow to cool and stir in the yoghurt. Serve chilled.

Easy calculation of calories

For easy calculation of calorific content, the average helping of the following is equal to approximately the calories given:

All-Bran	100
Apricots, tinned	150
Avocado (½)	100
Bacon, two rashers, fried	350
Baked beans	200
Beef, corned	250
Beef, roast	250
Beef, steak-and-kidney pudding	500
Beef, steak, grilled	325
Blancmange	150
Bournvita	50
Bream, red	100
Cheese, Camembert	100
Cheese, Cheddar	125
Cheese, Stilton	150
Cod, fried	250
Cornflakes	100
Custard, made with powder	100
Doughnuts	200
Duck, roast	350
Eggs, Scotch (1)	300
Eggs, scrambled (2)	200
Fruit jelly	100

Fruit salad	100
Gooseberry pie	300
Haddock, fried	300
Ham, boiled	400
Jam roll, baked	450
Kedgeree	150
Kipper (1)	200
Liver, fried	300
Luncheon meat	400
Mackerel, fried	300
Mince pies	150
Mussels	100
Orange (1)	50
Peach, fresh	50
Peas, fresh, boiled	50
Plaice, fried	400
Pork chop, grilled	600
Porridge	100
Potatoes, baked	100
Potatoes, chipped, fried	300
Potatoes, new, boiled	100
Rice Krispies	100
Sausages, pork, fried	200
Shepherd's pie	250
Shredded Wheat	100
Sole, fried	400
Spinach, boiled	25
Sponge pudding with syrup	400
Suet pudding	400
Toad-in-the-hole	500
Treacle tart	400
Turkey, roast	225
Vita-Weat	100
Welsh rarebit	300
Yoghurt, fruit	150

OTHER PAN BOOKS
AVAILABLE FROM PAN MACMILLAN

DR ROBERT C. ATKINS
ATKINS FOR LIFE   0 330 41846 7   £7.99
FIONA HUNTER & LYNNE ROBINSON
PILATES PLUS DIET   0 330 48954 2   £10.99
INNOCENT
STAY HEALTHY. BE LAZY.   0 7522 1595 7   £5.99

All Pan Macmillan titles can be ordered from our website,
www.panmacmillan.com, or from your local bookshop
and are also available by post from:

Bookpost, PO Box 29, Douglas, Isle of Man IM99 1BQ
Credit cards accepted. For details:
Telephone: 01624 677237
Fax: 01624 670923
E-mail: bookshop@enterprise.net
www.bookpost.co.uk

Free postage and packing in the United Kingdom

Prices shown above were correct at the time of going to press.
Pan.Macmillan reserve the right to show new retail prices on covers
which may differ from those previously advertised in the text
or elsewhere.